STROKE

By

Suzanne Smith R.N.

ISBN-13: 978-1976468032

ISBN-10: 1976468035

NOTICE

THIS BOOK IS INTENDED AS A HELPFUL
REFERENCE BOOK ONLY. NOT AS A MANUAL
FOR SELF-CARE OR TREATMENT, NOT AS A
MEDICAL GUIDE OR TREATMENT. IF YOU HAVE
MEDICAL PROBLEMS. PLEASE SEEK MEDICAL
ATTENTION, DO NOT WAIT. THE INFORMATION
HERE IS WRITTEN TO HELP YOU LEARN ABOUT
STROKES.

YOU ARE ENCOURAGED TO GET THE BEST CARE
POSSIBLE. THIS BOOK IS NOT A SUBSTITUTE FOR
YOUR PERSONAL NURSING OR MEDICAL CARE.
IF YOU HAVE QUESTIONS OR CONCERNS PLEASE
CONSULT WITH YOUR HEALTHCARE PROVIDER.

DEDICATION

To all who are seeking more information to achieve their best health possible. Those willing to make changes when necessary and are committed to working toward good health. **Good for you!**

Contents

Forward

After thirty years in healthcare, and many years in college, I never thought it would happen to me. STROKE. It sounded like a death sentence. After years of caring for stroke patients I was now one. I was the patient, with no health insurance. The Lutheran church loaned me a wheelchair; my nursing friends were dumb founded. I was the strong one, the go-to nurse. Now helpless, almost. Humbled, overwhelmed. My body would not behave as usual. I could not walk, read, or speak clearly. I slumped to the right- my affected side, and drooled. For three years a wheelchair was my home. My husband had died during that spring, and I was alone with my black lab.

Today I can walk over a mile and can communicate, sing, speak -even dance a little! So, this is a book of hope. Never give up hope. Never.

1 WHAT IS A STROKE?

Stroke is the top cause of death in the U.S. Sometimes it called a brain attack. In the hospital, we call a stroke a "CVA" which is a cerebral vascular accident.

Other names for stroke;

TIA Transient Ischemic Attack

CVA

Cerebral Vascular Accident

Brain Aneurysms

Brain Attack

What is stroke- what does it look like?

When oxygen rich blood is cut off from heathy brain tissue- the brain tissue dies. When that happens brain activity in the dead cells ends. The area of the body that had been controlled by those brain cells does not get the nerve messages from the dead tissue. Although the damage has occurred in the head, the effected part or parts of the body can be far from the head. The foot, the leg. Speech and sight, and swallowing are controlled by the brain. The brain is the command center for the entire body. Think about this illustration. My air conditioner works well and does a good job. But if my power goes out, and the air conditioner receives no energy, it is dead. It does not function. When my air conditioner's electric returns the unit will come alive. It will resume its activity- cooling restored.

But a stroke.........

There is a crucial time when a stroke is happening that medical care must be obtained quickly. Quick expert care may limit damage or possibly stop damage. Time is of the essence!

Regretfully, I hear so often that thoughtful intelligent people who suddenly suffer a sign of a possible stroke go to bed.' I thought I'd be better in the morning'.

Precious time is lost. Damage is continuing. What might have been a small stroke may now be a major stroke. Time matters.

REALLY

There are major types of stroke. They are different but the dangerous warning signs are the same. Small signs can mean big trouble.

TIA or Transient Ischemic Attack-Stroke

Transient means passing. The symptoms pass in a few minutes. This is an emergency -and may herald a major stroke may be on the way. Get medical attention now.

Ischemic Stroke

This is the most common. Something has blocked the flow of blood to heathy brain tissue. Sometimes the blockage occurs when an artery becomes too narrow for enough blood to pass through it. The narrowing occurs silently and is called stenosis. The buildup of cholesterol within the hollow interior causes narrowing and stiffening to the artery. As the buildup continues the flow of blood is obstructed. Then a blockage occurs.

This could be a blood clot, or a fat clot from another part of the body. When it travels to the brain it acts like a plug. On the other side of the plug the brain tissue is dying. Think of a garden hose with a cork in it. Within the hose there is water pressure, the hose is filled - pressure is building- but the cork is stopping you from watering the grass. Remember the old sea diver movies. The sea diver is down deep in the water -and something happens to his air hose. There is panic. Need to get the oxygen to the diver.

 As we get older our blood vessels can get plaque buildup and become stiff and like a hose that has been left in the sun for a couple of summers. Likewise, when a plug -a clot- obstructs the arteries of the brain or leading to the brain blood ceases to flow to the brain cells. Damage is occurring- death of cells will result. Stroke symptoms begin to occur. This is an emergency.

The more time, the more damage. Timely medical intervention may limit damage to the brain. *Seek medical attention at once.*

A place where this plug often occurs is the carotid arteries. These are the arteries which bring blood to your brain and are on the left and right side of your neck. There was an old saying in the hospital "hardening of the arteries softening of the brain". In some older people, the carotid arteries have a significant amount of build up within the vessels. The flow of oxygen rich blood slows down. Gradually. While this is occurring brain, cells are dying. And cognition and memory begin to slip. And continue to deteriorate. The examination of these arteries should be part of every older person's yearly examination. When the doctor puts his stethoscope of the side of your neck   (one side at a time) he is listening for a very distinctive sound.

If he has a concern, he will have an ultra-sound test done. If narrowing is discovered and   restored through surgery, good blood flow to the brain is restored. It is remarkable how the patient improves. The surgery is not without risk- speak to your doctor about it.

Hemorrhagic Stroke

Aneurysms are balloon-like bulges in an artery that can stretch and burst. Rupture, then hemorrhage.

Think of the garden hose- with a weak wall, and high pressure.

Pressure builds -and the bulging hose splits and bursts.

Water is pouring out. Water is not going where you intend it to go.

A Hemorrhagic stroke is a bleeding blood vessel in the brain. Cells are being starved of nourishing blood. The bleeding builds pressure within the brain- and damage is occurring. Symptoms are occurring. Medical help is needed at once.

Bottom line. When stroke symptoms occur, we must get medical attention immediately. Every minute counts.

Brain without oxygen

Hypoxia (hypo- means low oxygen) A reduction or less than adequate flow of oxygen rich blood to brain tissues.

After three minutes, there is damage- six to nine minutes the brain tissues deprived of oxygen are dying.

Timing really matters. Have a nudge or a concern go to the emergency room, now.

2 STROKE RISKS

There are things you can impact, and those you have no control over. Let us get the things out of the way that we have no control over. We are not going to fret over them, but simply be aware of them. Some you may be aware of, some not. Perhaps you know of others. Good for you. Let us press on!

Irregular Heart rhythm

An irregular heart rhythm can cause turbulence within the heart chambers. This turbulence can cause blood to clot. Then with the next beat the clot moves.

Problems with the heart valves

This causes the blood flowing through the heart chambers to experience turbulence. This can create blood clots.

Some **inherited risk factors** for stroke are genetics or ethnic family history. Blood vessels abnormalities present at birth, but not apparent until later.

African Americans have the highest incidence of stroke. The problem occurs because of high blood pressure which may be resistant to control with medicines. Genetic blood conditions like sickle cell anemia can also lead to strokes.

 Certain traditional ethnic diets are higher in salt and fat. Some individuals have a sensitivity to any extra salt in their diet. Sensitivity to salt is a symptom not to be ignored. As your heart pumps, it exerts pressure against the walls of the arteries. When our bodies swell from extra salt and the resulting retention of water the heart must work harder. Blood pressure goes up. Elevated blood pressure and ongoing high blood pressure exerts excessive ongoing pressure on all organs. This creates damage. The damage occurs silently but is very real. The first symptom may be a stroke. African -

Americans also have a higher incidence of diabetes and obesity which can contribute.

Hispanics, Native Americans, and Alaska Natives also have a higher incidence of stroke. Problems of high blood pressure, obesity and diabetes are also common in these groups, unfortunately.

A family history of stroke can put us at higher risk. This impacted me. But I never saw it coming. My maternal aunt and paternal grandfather both had strokes. My grandfather was 89 and died while building a rock wall for a neighbor in July. He worked until the day he died.

My stroke occurred when I was 58. I had a poor diet and was working seven days a week, a lot of stress. My aunt's stroke occurred when she was in her late sixties.

Age is also a risk factor. But young people can also have strokes. Young woman using birth control pills have an increased risk of stroke, especially if they also smoke. I have had stroke patients in their twenties.

Gender is a risk also. Men are more likely to have a stroke then women.

Pregnant women are more at risk.

Menopause is a risk factor.

Diabetes increases the risk of stroke and heart attack. Type 1 and type 2. High blood sugar levels damage blood vessels (you have blood vessels in your brain) and the nerves of your body. Damage to important nerves within your heart muscles can occur. In addition, nerves that control your blood vessels are also damaged. If you have diabetes it's important to control your blood sugar, your blood pressure and your weight. You will live longer and have more enjoyment in your life.

Certain blood disorders increase the risk of strokes.

TRAUMA

Head and neck injuries increase the risks.

A trauma to a limb, can create a blood clot- which can travel through your vessels to another part of your body. Think car accidents or falls.

Our long bones have marrow. Think of beef soup bones, and the fatty soft tissue inside the bone cavity.

If we suffer a break in a bone which has this reservoir of fatty tissue a piece can break off and enter the blood vessel. This a like a missile traveling in your blood. If this clump plugs up a blood vessel then the tissues beyond it are deprived of oxygen rich blood. Perhaps it will plug up a vein in a leg or go to the heart. Or go to the brain. A stroke can result.

Surgery of a serious nature carries risks. One of those risks is a stroke.

What are the things we can control?

Smoking reduces the oxygen your body is taking in. Your brain gets less oxygen. Smoking damages blood vessels and increases the buildup of plaques in blood vessels. Plaques which can break off. Causing a stroke. Exposure to secondhand smoke is almost as damaging.

Dehydration. The blood gets thicker. This increases the risk. Please stay hydrated. If your mouth is sticky, and your urine dark yellow chances are you are dehydrated. Check in at the emergency room to be safe.

The 1# Culprit is High Blood Pressure

High blood pressure is the *primary-that is number one* factor for stroke. Sometimes called hypertension. Also called the silent killer, because often the first symptom of high blood pressure is a stroke or heart attack, and sometimes death.

The heart is a double pump. One side pumps blood to the body the other side pumps blood to the lungs to get oxygen. It is a strong muscled organ.

As you know there are two numbers recorded when your blood pressure is measured.

The top number is the **systolic** (think sky)- this number records the degree of pressure of your blood pushing against your blood vessels when your heart pumps. Think PUSH.

The bottom number is the **diastolic** (think dirt-bottom). This number records the resting pressure of your blood -when, between beats, your heart rests.

Both these numbers are important.

Warning. Many of my home health patients had high blood pressure, and a home electronic monitor. Often, more often than you would think, they would measure their blood pressure and get an alarming high number. Or a weird number. Sometimes these numbers were given to their doctors, and doses of their high blood pressure medicine was changed. The punch line to this is – when I arrived at the home and measured with a manual cuff and my electronic cuff, I got different numbers, and had to call the doctor to report my findings.

The Electronic blood pressure cuffs are great, *but….*

Take your cuff with you when you go to the doctor and have them measure any difference in their equipment and yours. Next, and very importantly, *change the batteries every month.* Sooner if you get a strange reading. These cuffs don't last forever. Also, many fire departments and health departments will, as a courtesy, measure your blood pressure. Free. Just ask.

The older we get some of our blood vessels become coated with plaque, which narrows the path the blood must take. Narrow vessels higher pressure.

If we let food get the best of us and obesity sets in then the heart must pump blood through a lot of tissue.

One extra pound of fat requires seven (7) extra miles of blood vessels. So, ten extra pounds = 70 extra miles. Much more work for your heart. The heart must pump harder to meet the need.

A healthy adult heart beats roughly 100,800 times per day. (There are 1,440 minutes in a day, seventy beats a minute). A health adult heart weighs 8-10 ounce- what an industrious small organ! The heart does its best to keep up with changes in our bodies. If we continue to overeat, and obesity results, our heart may enlarge. This happens to try to accommodate the needs of the larger body mass.

An enlarged heart is called **Cardiomegaly**. Some people are born with this, others develop the condition. The heart muscles get larger and stiff. Sometimes there are no symptoms. But sometimes there are. Some symptoms are swelling of the ankles and shortness of breath with activity, or on exertion. This enlarged heart is at higher risk of developing blood clots. These blood clots can move through the heart and cause a stroke.

The enlarged heart condition can lead to the next stage- heart failure. This is also called **CHF Congestive heart failure**. The heart -a pump is doing the best it can- but it starts to fail. Working with a good cardiologist, getting on the right medications, achieving a healthy weight, and if directed a low salt intake, can allow the condition to stabilized. Lifestyle changes, especially quitting smoking and stopping bad eating habits, are so difficult. However, at some point, we all need to rein in our appetites to increase the quality of our health with the hope of lengthening our days.

When I worked on a cardiac care unit many of my patients were first time heart attack victims. They were very frightened and more than willing to change their lifestyle in hopes of surviving. Can we decide to make healthy changes before we get to the cardiac care unit? The choice is up to us.

Over the counter drugs

The U.S. Food and Drug Administration (FDA) is strengthening an existing label warning on non-aspirin non-steroidal anti-inflammatory drugs (NSAIDs). These increase the chance of a heart attack or stroke. NSAIDs are widely used to treat pain and fever from many different long- and short-term medical conditions such as arthritis, menstrual cramps, headaches, colds, and the flu. NSAIDs are available by prescription and over the counter (OTC). Examples of NSAIDs include ibuprofen, naproxen, diclofenac, and celecoxib.

The exception to this new finding is the old-time classic aspirin. Aspirin is a serious drug. And can cause bleeding if taken in excessive doses. Aspirin can also interact with other drugs- and can cause serious problems. I would direct you to call Poison Control in your state to learn the newest information about any drug, prescription, OTC, or herbal supplement.

Often, I have heard from highly intelligent people 'well I can buy this drug without a prescription so it's not really a drug'. Wrong.

Alcohol and illegal drug use also increase the risk of stroke. Even in young people. This includes cocaine, amphetamines, and other illegal drugs. It also includes using prescription drugs that are not yours or for reasons your doctor did not prescribe.

Little physical activity

Ok, I'll tell you another true story. A well-respected internal medicine doctor traveled by air for a trip which lasted a few hours. When he arrived at his cross-country destination he stood up and immediately had pain in his legs. His legs had numerous blood clots in his veins. There was a long hospital stay and thank God, he did not have a stroke. Blood clots within our circulatory system can lodge and block oxygen rich blood from reaching tissues. This can be the brain, heart, liver, kidney, wherever there are blood vessels.

So, what would have helped this good doctor to avoid the blood clots? MOVE. Our bodies were designed -were built- to be mobile! I've recently heard this ugly joke: A recliner and a remote control are a death sentence!

Lack of movement contributes to *many* serious problems.

If you have been in the hospital in the past few decades you may have been greeted by a cheerful nurse who entered your room a few times a day and said, 'let us go for a walk'. Ugh… There was great purpose for this. Movement -walking- discourages moisture setting in your lungs. Think avoiding pneumonia. Moving gets your circulation going -especially in your lower limbs. The heart pumps blood down to your feet -but muscle movement moves it back up the body. When we lay down -and stay still for extended periods of time- the blood pools in our lower extremities-

legs. This promotes bloods clots. Blood clots which can move.

Extended time sitting is unhealthy. We need to periodically get up and walk around. Wiggle our feet. I like an exercise – flexing my ankles -and pointing my toes to my nose. I do this every few minutes when I am somewhere and need to wait while sitting. This simple exercise help move blood back into circulation.

Taking a few walks, a day is better than sitting stationary for a week and jogging on Saturday. We need movement frequently. You doctor can direct you how to start an exercise plan.

Eating Poorly

Good food, simple foods are what we want. If you were building a new home would you go buy trash at the dump to build your dream house?

I would suggest you would get the best supplies you possibly could.

Our bodies only get the food we choose to eat. Our food sustains us, and rebuilds old and dying tissues, and keeps us strong. Helps us heal when sick or injured.

Good food would be eating fresh foods. Don't have sauces poured over your food. Put sauces on the side. Dip in to get a taste.

Your body will enjoy salads, vegetables, and lean cooked meats. Use olive oil, and a small amount of real butter. Try different spices -shun extra salt, and you will be on your healthy way!

Obesity

Extra weight lays a tremendous burden on your entire body. We weigh more and move less. We eat for the wrong reasons. Entertainment and recreation, emotional comfort, or because others are eating around us. Food is not the problem. Using food inappropriately is. Please ask your doctor what your ideal weight is. Make it your target. If possible, get a consultation with a dietician.

If you have diabetes go to a diabetic education class in your area. Your insurance may pay for it, and it will be time well spent.

About that belly

IMPORTANT BOOK: **Wheat Belly by William Davis MD.**

'Renowned cardiologist, William Davis, MD explains how eliminating wheat from our diets can prevent fat storage, shrink unsightly bulges, and reverse myriad health problems'.

My doctor referred me to this book.

Columbia University researchers discovered that people with abdominal obesity are at higher risk of ischemic stroke. **Abdominal obesity** carries the highest risk for people under age 65. Extra abdominal weight increases the already high risk for African Americans and Hispanics.

Cholesterol

We need cholesterol. Our bodies make it and we consume it. Each nerve of our body is protected with a myelin sheath- which is made from – you guessed it cholesterol! A buildup of this helpful insulator can be a problem. The blood vessels become lined and stiff with this substance. The vessel narrows. Blood is obstructed.

 Many people have a genetic tendency to have elevated cholesterol. They and their siblings and other blood related family members may have elevated levels. For these people, controlling cholesterol can be difficult. Their bodies may not respond as hoped to medications, or dietary changes.

Others of us are sensitive to our food intake of this fatty substance. With these folks a reduction in intake of cholesterol rich foods- fatty meats, cheeses, can reduce the blood level.

Recent viral or bacterial infections can cause vasculitis – inflation of blood vessels.

Vasculitis: inflamed blood vessels. Vessels become weak, increase in size, or can become narrower. They are inflamed and weakened. They can stretch or become completely blocked. This can happen anywhere in the body, the heart, the eyes, legs—and/or the brain.

There are rare conditions that can be the cause. Viral and bacterial infection can cause blood vessels to become inflamed. One of the infections which can cause this vasculitis is neuro-syphilis, a sexually transmitted disease. Another cause can be a spirochetal disease, Lyme neuroborreliosis. This is a rare form of Lyme disease, transmitted by ticks.

There are discussions about untreated oral infections creating vasculitis leading to stroke.

Allergic reactions or an adverse reaction to some medications can also be the cause.

There also can be auto-immune flare ups, (the body attacking itself) that can cause this inflammation.

Geography. The highest U.S. death rates from stroke occur in the southeastern United States.

Birth Control Pills and other hormones increase the risk of stroke in all ages especially in smokers.

Lack of adequate sleep

Stress

Depression

Sleep. Your body needs time to rest and repair. Our minds need sleep to sort out our experiences and concerns. Some hormones are active while we sleep. Adequate sleep is not a luxury it is a necessity.

We cannot be all things to all people. WE must care for our own needs. We were designed to rest and renew. Setting aside one day a week to rest will renew your body and spirit.

Having a bedtime ritual- bath/shower, brush teeth. Quiet room to sleep in. Shut off the TV. Sleep in comfortable night clothes.

Still need help. Speak to your doctor.

Stress, we all have it. Some have more than their share. Always connected and available means we are always at work.

Depression. Most people at some time in their lives suffer from depression. Perhaps from the loss of a loved one. Sometimes there is a genetic predisposition to depression. Sometimes it is something physical going on and depression is a result. Please talk to your regular doctor. And Do not hesitate to tell him how you are really feeling. He can offer many kinds of real help.

Inflammation Today there is a lot of medical discussion suggesting there may be a connection between inflammation in the body and stroke. Studies are under way now. It suffices to say that chronic infection such as an oral infection emits the chemicals of inflammation and infection throughout your body.

More information is needed on this problem- but cleaning up oral infections and any chronic infection will be helpful for the entire body.

Ok, Ok! You are saying 'enough already!'

Skim through the list -circle what you have that you can't impact on those things you were born with. Then check those things you have that you can change.

Information is power. Plan to improve what you can control. Are you overweight? Well, my friend you did not get heavy overnight. Anyway, it's impossible to make a huge change in a small amount of time.

But you can identify what needs to improve. Have a meaningful discussion with your doctor. And the two of you plan and set goals.

Every journey begins with the first step. Please decide to get as healthy as you can.

3 Stroke danger signs

F.A.S.T.

F face- smile please- is your smile crooked ? Is you face drooping?

A Arms – raise your arms, is one arm weak? Un-able to raise? Or does it bend down? Weakness?

S Speech Is speech slurred? Or are they having trouble understanding?

T Time if you or the person you are with to call 911 immediately.

Remember a stroke is a brain attack. The brain is the command center of the body. When a stroke occurs the signal to part of the body is interrupted. Let us look at some of these signs. All the items on this list are danger signs. Although some may seem more serious than others. They are all serious and need medical attention quickly.

DANGER SIGNS OF STROKE

- Sudden severe headache
- Numbness of the leg, arm, hand, face-especially on one side
- Facial droop-drooping smile
- Slurred speech
- Difficulty swallowing
- Trouble speaking
- Trouble understanding
- Confusion
- New difficulty seeing in one or both eye
- Seeing double
- Sudden weakness anywhere in the body-arms, legs, hands, etc.
- New difficulty walking
- Loss of coordination
- Loss of balance
- Dizziness
- Word searching
- Memory lapses

- **Change in personality.**
- **Feeling 'different'**

If you have any of these -even one sign please get medical care quickly.

Do not drive yourself to the emergency room. Many times, horrible accidents occur when a good driver drives themselves to the emergency room. Only to have and accident, and sometimes lives are lost.

Time is important. Deprived of oxygen rich blood, in three minutes the brain cells are being damaged.

Six to nine minutes there is brain tissue death.

With quick medical care, we can hope for some damage being reversed, additional damage stopped, and a good prognosis for recovery. There are many facets to the process of a stroke. Where it is, what kind it is, and how quickly care is received. Many variables – some can be controlled, some not.

Give yourself the best opportunity for recovery. Get good help fast.

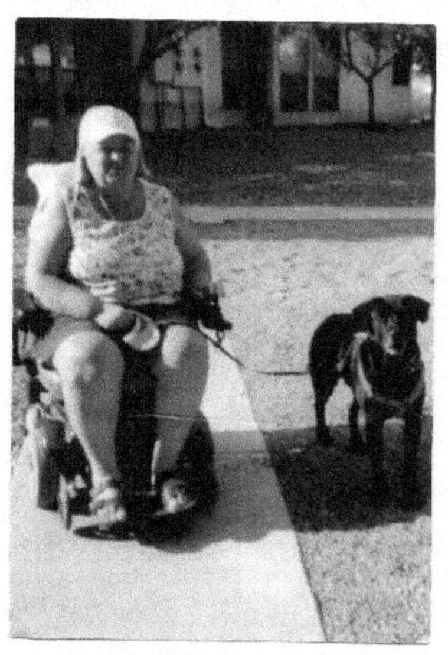

4 Recovering

There are many aspects of recovery- each stroke is unique, just as each person is unique. So, it's not one size fits all. But there *are* some common elements.

First the doctors will want to discover *why* you had a stroke. This will involve *CT scans* (computed tomography) and *MRIs* (magnetic resonance imaging). These are scans-a type of ex-rays of the brain. They do not hurt-but may require a trip into a narrow tunnel-while the scanning machine travels around the patient. There is a bit of noise- things are close. But it does not last long and gives a lot of information.

Computed Tomography Arteriogram and Magnetic Resonance Arteriogram: these scans will focus on the arteries within the brain.

These tests point to the location of the damage and the extent of the damage to the brain.

Carotid Ultrasound will be done to find out if your carotid arteries are blocked or narrow and if they contributed to the stroke. A smooth plastic wand is smoothed over the sides of your neck -while sound waves create an image of the blood vessels.

Angiography. This test requires a thin wire passed in to your body at the groin then up through the carotid arteries – a dye is released and the flow of the fluid can be seen on a screen and recorded.

An EKG is done to see what rhythm the heart is in. An irregular heartbeat can contribute to the formation of blood clots.

Echocardiography is a painless wand passed over the heart which sends radio waves and can record the presence of abnormal valves and clots within the heart.

There will be blood tests.

As you see there will be an investigation-what caused the stroke, where the damage is and what type of damage is there.

Attitude. The attitude of the stroke patient and the people close to them is a major factor in recovery. Family members and friends please be very patient. Your loving and compassionate support and encouragement are essential to recovery and survival.

The person with a stroke may have a difficult time with depression, communication, eating, mobility, and knowing where they fit into the world now. Love and acceptance are strong medicine. Please hang in there.

The road to recovery begins when you enter a hospital with a neurologist or better yet a hospital which either specializes in neurology or a specialized neurology hospital. Then you will know that everyone who you encounter is educated in helping with unique and specific needs.

A thorough assessment is the beginning. Ongoing assessments will be needed and must continue to see if there is additional damage. Progress is measured and discussed with the patient and family. There will be necessary adjustments to the plan of care as conditions change. All this while preexisting conditions are managed.

A physiatrist this is in MD or DO who specializes in rehabilitation. These are experts on movement. An evaluation by a neurologist, a physiatrist and a speech therapist is needed. These three are needed for a thorough evaluation. Their recommendations are the starting point of your recovery. A speech therapist or a speech pathologist will assess the ability of speaking and understanding language, memory, and the cognitive status. ALSO, *and very importantly* they will assess the ability to swallow.

A physical therapist will follow the orders of the physiatrist and neurologist to work on restoring mobility.

An occupational therapist will work with the patient to learn how to resume those activities needed to care for oneself. Cooking, dressing, putting on shoes, getting in and out of the car. All this and much more may be needed to be re-learned.

A counselor is ever so helpful for the patient and the family and friends. There are a lot of changes, and new things to learn. Perhaps even new responsibilities. The counselor can help with coping skills, resources like support groups, connecting with home health services, and staying on course with encouragement. A counselor will help all involved with understanding the emotional challenges of a stroke. Often a stroke will cause emotions to be very fragile-with crying easily, struggling with depression, and frustration for all involved.

Your spiritual counselor, pastor, or rabbi will be a precious link to healing. A stroke totally humbled me-I lost hope. But found it with good counsel.

****

Now I want to tell you a story. An athletic lady in her early sixties, a golfer, had a mild stroke. She was in a major hospital. She was talking and had some weakness on one side. She had every reason to be hopeful of recovery. And her husband was at her side.

She could talk and eat independent of assistance. So, no consultation with the speech therapist was ordered.

Two days after her stroke her husband reported that she had a cold.

Three days later she died. She was inhaling some of her food, and because of the stroke she lost the sensation of food going into her lungs. A swallowing study done by a speech therapist would have caught that and she would have had treatment and teaching on swallowing and gone on to play more golf.

***

Rehabilitation will begin when the patient is medically stable. Usually within a few days. At first the rehab may be within the hospital setting. Then a patient may be moved to a rehabilitation unit outside of the hospital. These facilities should continue with the needed therapies as prescribed by the doctors.

Speech therapists, physical therapists, occupational therapists, counselors, and the dietician should all be on board with the patient's unique needs and goals. Within these units the patients preexisting conditions need to be managed well. Blood pressure and blood sugar should be under control. Family and friends need to continue to visit and support and encourage the patient.

The nurses and care staff should be experienced in caring for patients with a stroke. They as the other professionals should be available to teach patient, family, and friends how best to walk through the rehabilitation process. Visiting often and asking questions can help maintain good care. And the value to the patient is beyond measure.

There will be changes – they may be long or short term. Celebrate every inch of progress.

You may even receive rehabilitation services in your home. A Registered Nurse familiar with stroke recovery, with a physical therapist, the speech therapist, an occupational therapist may come to your home. You may also receive the care of an aide, who will tidy up your home and help you bath. You may need medical equipment. Hospital bed, bed side toilet, diapers, special spoon and fork, delivered meals-your nurse will be your case manager, and will work with the other disciplines to provide a safe home environment to help your recovery.

A social worker will help you secure services you may need. These can be special transportation and shopping services. She may avail herself as a supportive counselor, also. The social worker in home health can assist with resources within the community.

Do not lose track of your spiritual counselor. This is all work. You will want someone to talk to you can trust.   Stay encouraged!

■■

My major stroke in 09' took my ability to understandably communicate verbally or in written form. It was bewildering to slur my words. People could not understand me when I spoke. I typed what I was trying to express and what was on the screen was different. It was immensely scary when my body would not behave as I was accustomed. The right side of my body was very weak.

I was drooling while awake. I could not control my bladder. And all this is the short list.

I was overwhelmed. Widowed and alone. But I had a great dog-a black lab who rose to the occasion and was a wonderful helper.

As a nurse, I had cared for many stroke patients-but now it was me.

Today I live with my service dog, but no additional help. My speech and written communication have returned. I was in a wheelchair for three years- now I can walk a mile. No cane, no walker. BUT there was a lot of work. Painful baby steps at first. But always, always pressing on.

To me recovering is rather like preparing for the Olympics. You get up early, you challenge yourself, you press on daily. You have your personal goals, and good healthy food. Always staying hydrated-even if you lose control of your bladder often.

My rehab started by going to Silver Sneakers at the YMCA. My exercises were done while in my electric wheelchair. Everyone was truly kind.

Every day I challenged myself -as did my dearest friends, to press on. I started eating healthier food. While I was in the wheelchair my entertainment was eating. I had gained over eighty pounds. The extra weight made my recovery more difficult, more painful and lengthy then it would have been.

 It was very much like preparing for an Olympic event. But the gold medal I wanted was to walk and talk clearly.

It took two years to lose eighty pounds. Gradually, I grew stronger and got my balance restored.

Major Points in Recovering:

Seek the best rehabilitation care you can get.

Physiatrist, Physical Therapist, Speech Therapist, Occupational Therapist, Registered Nurse.

Supporting and compassionate friends, family, Pastor or Rabbi.

Seek the best general physical health-good heart health and blood pressure, great blood sugars.

Set goals-to restore what was damaged-perhaps to be better than you were prior to the event.

Look forward! Like an athlete looking to a big competition-the best healthy diet, exercise, and rest. Focus, endurance, and hope.

You can't afford to be detoured by negative thoughts! Eyes on the prize! Avoid negative thoughts like the flu!

You are winning if you do not quit.

Measure and record your progress.

Make a daily schedule – and give yourself one day of rest every week.

Develop situational awareness. Use ramps, handrails, good shoes. *NO THROW RUG IN THE HOME.*

Keep good company- encouragers.

Don't avoid fluids to limit urination. Wear pads- save your kidneys.

Get out of the house- avoid seclusion. You need community and sunshine.

Give yourself healthy rewards. Flowers, county fair, visit friends, music.

Think of 'The Little Engine That Could';

___I think I can, I think I can I think I can and God will carry me through!___

Every stroke is different.

Every person is unique.

Never stop trying.

Never give up hope.

EVERY DAY do something towards your recovery.

Review the resources I have added. Get the best help you can. Keep trying, keep working. Do not give up!

A stroke is not the end- it's a new beginning!

STROKE References & Resources

Contact for Suzanne Smith R.N.:
old.nurse@yahoo.com

Chapter 1 What is a stroke?

Wikipedia contributors. *Hypoxia* (medical). Wikipedia, The Free Encyclopedia. September 14, 2017, 10:58 UTC. Retrieved from: https://en.wikipedia.org/w/index.php?title=Hypoxia_(medical)&oldid=800572028.

Zeratsky, Katherine R.D., L.D. Oct. 2014 Healthy Lifestyle, Mayo Clinic. Nutrition and healthy eating, Nutrition-wise blog. *Like adults, children are eating too much salt.* Retrieved from: http://www.mayoclinic.org/healthy-lifestyle/nutrition-and-healthy-eating/expert-blog/children-eating-too-much-salt/bgp-20113918

Chapter 2 Stroke Risks

U.S. Department of Health & Human Services. (2017). *Who Is at Risk for a Stroke?* National Institutes of Health, NHLBI January 27, 2017 National Institutes of Health. Retrieved from: https://www.nhlbi.nih.gov/health/health-topics/topics/stroke/atrisk

National Institutes of Health, U.S. Department of Health & Human Services. (2017) *Description of High Blood Pressure. Health Information for the Public, Sept. 2015* Retrieved from: https://www.nhlbi.nih.gov/health/health-topics/topics/hbp

Magnant, Dr. Joseph .M.D. February 15, 2016 *One Pound of Fat = 7 Miles of Blood Vessels!* Vein Specialists at Royal Palm Square1510 Royal Palm Square Blvd.Suite 101Fort Myers, Florida 33919 P. 239.694.VEIN (8346) www.WeKnowVeins.com

Cardiovascular Surgery of Southern Nevada (Sept. 2013). *How Many Times Does Your Heart Beat Per Day?* Cardiovascular Surgery of Southern Nevada 5320 S. Rainbow Blvd. t: 1.800.200.2128 Suite 282 Las Vegas, NV 89118 Retrieved from: http://www.cvsurgnv.com/how-many-times-does-your-heart-beat-per-day/

Dougherty, Matthew (Aug.2003) *Stroke Study Finds Abdominal Obesity a Stroke risk factor/Rising obesity rates puts younger people at risk.* In VIVO , Columbia University. Retrieved from: http://www.cumc.columbia.edu/publications/in-vivo/Vol2_Iss13_aug18_03/stroke.html

Davis, William, MD (2011). *Wheat Belly: Lose the Wheat, Lose the Weight, and Find Your Path Back to Health*. Retrieved from: http://www.wheatbellyblog.com/

Mayo Clinic Staff (Jan. 2017). *Enlarged Heart, Patient Care & Health Information, Diseases & Conditions Enlarged heart* The Mayo Clinic 480-301-8000 13400 E. Shea Blvd. Scottsdale, AZ 85259. Retrieved from: http://www.mayoclinic.org/diseases-conditions/enlarged-heart/symptoms-causes/dxc-20305824

FDA. (2016). FDA Drug Safety Communication: *FDA strengthens warning that non-aspirin nonsteroidal anti-inflammatory drugs (NSAIDs) can cause heart attacks or stroke.*For More Info 855-543-DRUG (3784) and press 4 Retrieved from: druginfo@fda.hhs.gov

Phillips, David B.Ph.D. (n.d.) *What is peripheral neuropathy?* Retrieved from: http://www.peripheralneuropathytreatments.com/therebuilder.htm

Phone: 951-303-3471 9-5 Pacific Time

Email: info@peripheralneuropathytreatments.com Frequency Rising 5658 Antigua Blvd. San Diego, California 92124

National Kennedy Shiver National Institute of Child Health and Human Development- US Department of Health and Human Services NIH, (Aug 2012). *What causes stroke?* Centers for Disease Control and Prevention. Stroke. Retrieved from: http://www.cdc.gov/stroke/

National Institute of Neurological Disorders and Stroke. (2012). *Stroke: Hope through research.* Retrieved from: http://www.ninds.nih.gov/disorders/stroke/detail _stroke.htm

Rupprecht, Tobias A; Koedel, Uwe; Fingerle, Volker; Pfister, Hans-Walter (2008). *The Pathogenesis of Lyme Neuroborreliosis: From Infection to Inflammation.* Molecular Medicine. 14 (3–4): 205–212. PMC 2148032 . PMID 18097481. doi:10.2119/2007-00091.Rupprecht .

Chapter 4 STROKE danger signs

National Institutes of Health, U.S. Department of Health & Human Services (2017). *What Are the Signs and Symptoms of a Stroke?* Retrieved from: https://www.nhlbi.nih.gov/health/health-topics/topics/stroke/signs

American Stroke Association (n.d.). *F.A.S. T.* Retrieved from:

http://www.strokeassociation.org/STROKEORG/WarningSigns/Stroke-Warning-Signs-and-Symptoms_UCM_308528_SubHomePage.jsp

Chapter 5 RECOVERING

National Institutes of Health, (2017). *Life After a Stroke.* Retrieved from: https://www.nhlbi.nih.gov/health/health-topics/topics/stroke/lifeafter

Mayo Clinic. (May 2017). *Stroke rehabilitation: What to expect as you recover.* Retrieved from: http://www.mayoclinic.org/diseases-conditions/stroke/in-depth/stroke-rehabilitation/ART-20045172

Piper,Watty, Munk,Arnold,(1930).*The Little Engine That Could.* Published by Platt & Munk

ABOUT THE AUTHOR

Suzanne Smith R.N., born in Philadelphia, Pa. and has enjoyed serving others with tender nursing care and strong patient advocacy. She came up through the ranks- first as a nursing assistant- then an LPN, then a Registered Nurse. She earned a CPHQ- Certified Professional in Healthcare Quality in 2004. A graduate of the University of the State of New York- Regents College, Albany, NY. and Pima Community College, Tucson, Arizona- Honors and Phi Theta Kappa. She has had chaplaincy training and is a Parish Nurse. A lifelong student of theology -and a Bible teacher.

Smith has been honored by Congressmen and other community leaders for work with the senior citizens. Smith has worked in the Medical departments of two HMOs in the role of Utilization Review, Prior Authorization, Concurrent Review, Quality Assurance, Case Manager/Discharge Planner/ Quality Improvement. She also worked in those roles within a private hospital and Home Health. She has been a board member of the United Way- Healthcare Allocations committee, served in the Red Cross, and numerous other volunteer positions.

Other books by Suzanne;

- **INTERNATIONAL HEALTH SCOUT**
-
- **SALT** where it is and what it does.

- **Gorilla Healthcare Skills** getting better healthcare

- **Nurse In my Pocket** avoiding. medical errors

An adventure, non- fiction book

- **CROPDUSTER"S WIFE**

All on Amazon and Kindle

Healthscout.mum@gmail.com

Thank you for reading my book.

Sincerely,

Sue